HOW I CURED
MY A-FIB

by

Jay Clarke

CONTENTS

Medical Disclaimer

It is an absolute condition of sale/use that you accept the following terms and conditions

The content of this book is for information only and is not a substitute for qualified medical advice. No person should make any medical decisions based on information presented here-in without first consulting a qualified medical practitioner.

The content of this book should not be used for any diagnostic or treatment purposes.

If you are suffering or think you are suffering from any medical condition you should seek immediate medical attention

Whilst reasonable efforts have been made to check the accuracy of the information contained herein the authors will not be held liable for errors of omissions that may be found.

Information in this book should never be used in place of qualified medical advice.

The author does not specifically endorse or recommend any of the treatments or course of actions within this book and you agree they will not be held liable in any way for any action or decision taken in relation to the information in this book.

ABOUT A-FIB

For anyone suffering from the challenging and unpredictable heart condition, atrial fibrillation, I hope my story gives hope. As a disclaimer I would like to state that this book is in no way designed to substitute for proper medical care, nor should you try the strategies within it without proper medical supervision. This is merely the story, from a non-medical perspective of how I managed to cure my own a-fib.

The medical profession is very reluctant to declare any condition 'cured' preferring instead to use the vague term 'remission'. This always implies the possibility that the condition is going to come back. If you had been knocked over by a car and survive, doctors don't say you are in remission from being knocked over by cars! Instead, I prefer to use the word cure – as that is what I believe I am.

How do I know? Well I have gone from runs of a-fib every single day to no episodes at all for a considerable length of time, several years in fact. I would call that evidence of a cure. I take no a-fib medications, nor have I had surgery. What I have tried to do is methodically figure out what was causing this crazy arrhythmia and fix it myself. The road was long and involved a lot of research and experimentation, but the prize was totally worth the time and effort.

At this point I would like to say that there are different 'flavours' of a-fib. Firstly, there is a-fib caused by underlying structural changes in the heart which can include valve problems or problems with the physical structure of the heart itself. This is sometimes known as valvular a-fib.

Secondly, there is what doctors used to call 'lone' a-fib, when a-fib occurs in structurally normal hearts with no apparent risk factors. This type of a-fib usually occurs in younger people and this is the type of atrial fibrillation I was diagnosed with. This is often the type that creates the greatest challenge for doctors as it requires a fair bit of detective work in order to figure out what exactly is initiating these episodes. As this variety is often considered more benign than valvular a-fib, sometimes little effort is put into finding the cause and patients are told 'to live with it'.

There is also atrial fibrillation which is caused by lifestyle factors. It it well known by A&E doctors that a-fib can be brought on by binge drinking, overindulgence in food and indeed by stress. In fact, these triggers for a-fib are so common that they are even given a name 'holiday heart'. Obesity has finally been recognised as another factor in the initiation of a-fib and surprisingly a-fib can also be initiated by stomach problems. I'll go through some of the things which I found could trigger a-fib later in this book.

Obviously, if you have an underlying structural heart problem, you are not going to be able to fix it yourself, but under the supervision of your doctor you may find many of the strategies which I have listed here effective. I stress, under the supervision of your doctor – never stop taking medication or begin supplementation or any other significant lifestyle change without the agreement of your doctor. However, some factors such as losing even 5% of your body weight (if overweight of course!) can cause significant improvements to the structure of the heart. I did a lot of research into how excess weight contributed to a-fib when searching for my cure.

If you have no structural heart disease or have been told by doctors that there is no apparent reason for your a-fib episodes I hope you will find some useful information in this book. It is incredibly frustrating to be told by experts that there is no explanation for your condition, particularly with all the advances in science and medicine recently. When I was diagnosed, I was relatively young with no known health problems, and all the doctors could do was scratch their heads. I was told that what I had was very unusual for my age but was not considered life threatening. The condition was likely to be progressive, and if it did progress there were many things they could do to control it, but they had absolutely no idea why I had developed a-fib in the first place!

I'm the sort of person who likes to deal in absolutes and answers and this state of uncertainty caused a lot of unnecessary anxiety and fear. A-fib was already causing a great deal of chaos in my life, I had suddenly gone from someone who was carefree to someone living with the constant threat of admission to a cardiology ward. So, I started to look for my own answers.

I asked specialists, I read medical paper after medical paper, examined the latest research, joined forums and swapped stories with other patients. I found a lot of other people who had managed to cure themselves of a-fib but also that there was no magic cure which worked for everyone. It was very much a case of finding out what works for the individual.

Some of the greatest wisdom I came across came not from Western medicine but from the Chinese. In the West, we tend to treat a-fib as a stand-alone disease, whereas in the East a-fib is considered a symptom of an imbalance in the body. If we can figure out what is out of balance, then we can take steps to remedy it and return the body to total health. Whilst that sounds simplistic when you think about the concept it makes perfect sense.

I believe that everything happens for a reason. Being fobbed off by a doctor saying 'it's just one of those things' or 'a-fib is a disease of the aging heart' doesn't address any of the underlying factors which contribute to a-fib. A-fib doesn't occur without a cause, whether that cause is structural problems in the heart, nutritional deficiencies, excess weight, dietary factors, alcohol, systemic diseases or a myriad of other factors.

Being told a-fib isn't life threatening isn't much consolation when each attack brings intense anxiety and complete disruption to your life. Unless a physician has actually experienced the misery of a wildly unpredictable heartbeat, the physical and mental symptoms which attacks cause they may have little understanding of the impact a-fib actually has on your day to day wellbeing.

As such, doctors often focus on treating the symptoms rather than the root cause. In their defence, a-fib is the most common arrythmia a general practitioner will see, and every individual has their own underlying reasons for developing it. But, with a-fib a little detective work pays dividends, so if your doctor hasn't already referred you for a full work up and a visit to a cardiologist to investigate further don't be fobbed off with "it's just one of those things". At the very minimum you need to know your CHA_2DS_2-VASc score which calculates your risk of stroke, and have an ECG and an echocardiogram to look at the structure and size of the heart.

If your a-fib is caused by structural heart problems, it is unlikely that you will be able to make it go away by itself without first correcting the underlying cause. Nevertheless, the strategies in this book may improve your condition considerably by reducing the burden on your heart and generally improving your lifestyle factors.

For many of us however, a-fib is more of a disease of lifestyle than of the heart itself. High blood pressure, high blood sugar, carrying too many pounds, a poor diet, stress and vitamin and mineral deficiencies all take their toll on the heart and make it more likely to develop a-fib.

In the past few years, research has confirmed this hypothesis and has shown that intensive lifestyle intervention can not only reduce the severity and number of episodes of a-fib a person suffers, but it can also make it go away altogether. The cure for some people could be as simple as losing 10% of their body weight or an average of 36lbs for people who are very overweight and keeping it off.

Of course though, not everyone who has a-fib is overweight, just as not everyone who is overweight develops a-fib. How irritable the atria are is highly variable from person to person, some people can have numerous lifestyle risk factors and never develop any form of arrythmia whilst others suffer from the most irritable and bad tempered atria and suffer constantly from skipped beats and episodes of a-fib.

I mentioned earlier that a-fib is the most common arrythmia seen in general practice and it is estimated that somewhere around 1% and 6% of adults have the condition. In fact it is thought that 1 in 4 of us will have at least one atrial fibrillation episode in our lifetime, which is an awful lot of GP consultation hours taken up with this pesky complaint.

With this in mind, your GP may not have the time and resources to dig down into exactly WHY this is happening to you. They will probably refer you to a cardiologist who will run some tests, check the size, function and rhythm of your heart, check your bloods and evaluate your stroke risk. They may start you on some medication and blood thinners, but they probably don't have the time to figure out all the contributory factors. They will treat the symptoms but not the root cause.

Educating yourself about the condition and what you can do to improve or even cure it will not only take much of the fear out of the diagnosis, it will also allow you to regain a sense of control. A-fib striking out of the blue can be terrifying, something medical professionals sometimes underestimate when talking to patients.

For the vast majority of patients, a-fib is not considered life threatening, it is more life disrupting. It can have some nasty complications, the chances of which can be reduced considerably with the right treatment. There are procedures which offer a good chance of a cure and it is perfectly possibly to live a full and a long life even in permanent a-fib.

Jay Clarke

What Is A-fib?

A-fib is an arrythmia, a disruption to the regular beating of the heart. It is a problem with the electrical system which tells your heart when and how quickly to beat. It is not a heart attack - that involves a blockage of the plumbing of the heart (arteries and veins).

In a-fib the signals which are sent to the heart to keep it in a steady rhythm go haywire and the atria, the top part of the heart suddenly start to fibrillate very quickly. Whilst this sounds quite dangerous it really isn't as bad as it sounds as it is the bottom part of the heart, the ventricles which are responsible for pushing most of the blood around your body. So, you probably aren't at risk of keeling over, but the heart will be working around 20% less effectively than it normally does.

Whilst most people can continue normal activities during an attack, you might feel more tired than usual. Obviously if you have an existing condition such as heart failure that is making the heart pump less effectively than normal, then you will feel this more acutely. Speak to your doctor who will advise you on a safe level of activity and what you should do if you feel an attack coming on.

A-fib can be divided into three categories depending on how long each attack lasts and whether or not the heart converts back to normal rhythm on its own. Episodic a-fib, also known as paroxysmal a-fib lasts less than 48 hours and the heart converts back to its normal rhythm naturally. It may last for only a few seconds or for several hours.

Persistent a-fib is of longer duration, 7 days or more and often requires some form of intervention to get the heart to convert back to normal rhythm. This is known as a cardioversion and can be done with either drugs or a short electric shock to the chest in the outpatient department.

If your attack has lasted more than 24-48 hours you will usually be given a scan and/or some blood thinning medicine before undergoing a cardioversion. This is to stop any blood clots which may have formed in the heart being dislodged during the procedure.

Lastly, permanent a-fib is where a-fib becomes the normal rhythm of the heart. Permanent a-fib is unlikely to convert back to sinus (natural) rhythm spontaneously, but many people can and do live life to the full in permanent a-fib.

Luckily medical science has moved on a great deal when it comes to this arrythmia and there are treatments such as ablation which can stop the heart from misfiring. Whilst this works most effectively for episodic a-fib, it can also work for permanent a-fib too.

What Actually Happens During A-fib?

A-fib starts with an irritable focus within the hearts electrical system. Imagine electrical current passing through several circuits in a regular and orderly manner. That is how your heart normally beats, in a rhythm known as sinus rhythm. Then one day, one of these circuits decides to act up. Instead of passing the current through smoothly it decides to throw a hissy fit and hurl the current in all directions. When this happens during an a-fib attack, the atria start to fibrillate wildly at 300-600 cycles per minute.

Luckily, the heart has a built-in fail-safe mechanism. As we discussed earlier the ventricles - the lower part of the heart are responsible for most of the work in pushing blood around your body. When you feel your pulse at rest when your heart is beating normally it is usually around 60-100 beats per minute.

Now, consider that the atria are fibrillating at 300-600 beats per minute, if every single one of those beats were passed down to the ventricles you would have a pulse of over 300 bpm. At those rates your heart couldn't pump enough blood around your body to keep you alive and would soon wear itself out trying. So, the heart has a fail-safe node which only passes some of those beats down to the ventricles. As only certain impulses pass down, you get the typically irregularly irregular pulse which is indicative of a-fib.

Some people don't feel a-fib at all and it is only noticed when a doctor checks their pulse or they have an ECG. Other people (like me!) notice every single second of it. It may feel like your heart is hammering, skipping beats, speeding up, slowing down and is completely devoid of any sort of rhythm. You might feel a little tired or light-headed and feel the need to pee more than usual.

It is very common to feel fear when you are having an a-fib attack, but adrenaline just serves to make the heart faster and more ir-ritable. As you grow more used to a-fib and you realise that you have survived every other attack and you will survive this one you will learn to relax, which itself can help to bring you out of an attack.

It was a long time before I was able to sleep whilst I was in a-fib but invariably if I dropped off to sleep, I would awake in the night in normal rhythm or just about to convert to it. This became such a regular occurrence, I no longer worried about going to sleep during an attack. In fact I never once awoke in the morning still in a-fib, my attacks would always convert some time in the early hours.

Why Is It Important That I Get my A-fib Treated?

Left untreated a-fib can have some pretty nasty complications. Luckily, treatment can prevent and reduce the risk of them happening to you. Even if you only have occasional episodes it is important to speak to your doctor about your options for treatment, in particular anti-coagulation (thinning the blood).

The major and pretty devastating side-effect of a-fib is that it can increase your risk of having a stroke. Because the atria are essentially jiggling about very fast during an attack, blood can pool and stagnate, causing a clot. If this blood clot breaks loose (this can happen when the heart starts to pump normally again) it can travel to different parts of the body, such as the brain. Taking blood thinners will reduce the chance of this happening.

Different patients have different risk factors for stroke. Doctors use a formula known as the CHA_2DS_2-VASc score to work out your odds of having a stroke. This does not mean you are going to have a stroke, but it can help your doctor to decide whether you need to go on blood thinners.

Many people who have a-fib will never experience a stroke, whereas people who don't have a-fib do. There is no crystal ball to decide which patients will have a stroke but there are several known risk factors which increase the chances.

High blood pressure, diabetes, previous stroke or TIA, advancing age and being a female are some of the risk factors which doctors use to calculate your risk. Depending on your score they might recommend a blood thinner. Low risk patients may not require any form of anti-coagulation but for most patients one of the newer blood thinners will work extremely effectively.
At one time, doctors thought it was the length of a-fib episodes which determined which patients were at risk of a clot. It takes a certain amount of time for blood to clot and 48 hours was believed to be the magic number.

Newer thinking is that is isn't the amount of time you spend in a-fib but the company that a-fib keeps that provides the real risk of stroke in much the same way as certain risk factors increase the chances of a heart attack. Therefore, it pays to work on as many modifiable risk factors that you may have, losing weight, getting blood pressure under control and keep blood sugar normal.

Obviously, there is not much you can do about getting older or being female but intensive lifestyle modification has been proved to reduce or even eliminate a-fib altogether.

Conventional Treatments For A-fib

Doctors generally take a two-fold approach to treating a-fib conventionally, blood thinners if needed and drugs to either control the rate or the rhythm of the heart. For many years drugs were the first line of treatment but newer, minimally invasive procedures such as ablation have been developed which are proving to be extremely effective in both the short and long term eradication of the condition.

It is often said that 'a-fib begets a-fib' meaning that the longer the heart stays in a-fib and the more attacks you have, it becomes easier for an a-fib attack to start. A-fib remodels the heart over time making an a-fib attack more likely. However not everyone who has a-fib progresses further, my attacks stayed stable for years and never ran over the 24-hour mark. However it is generally accepted that a-fib should be quite aggressively treated from the start and ablations rather than being the last resort they used to be, are now the first line treatment in many cases.

Over the 20 or so years since catheter ablation for a-fib has been practiced, it has evolved and improved immensely. During the procedure, which is often done on a day case basis, a small catheter is fed into the heart and burns or freezes the irritable tissues which are causing the problem. In many cases, the troublesome foci are located around the entrance to the pulmonary veins. The scar tissue created by the procedure creates a sort of roadblock which prevents the irritable tissue from initiating atrial fibrillation.

The success rates for the procedure can be in the region of 95% depending on the skill of the operator and the type of a-fib. Episodic atrial fibrillation responds best to ablation, however there may be a need for a touch up procedure or even several touch ups to ensure all the potential trouble spots are gone. For persistent a-fib, the success rates are lower but may still be in the region of 50%.

Ablations, like any invasive procedure are not without risk. Even though the risks are relatively small for most people, things can and occasionally do go wrong. In my opinion (and I stress this is a non-medical one) intensive lifestyle modification and elimination or reduction of risk factors could be as effective as an ablation depending on the cause of your a-fib. I am not trying to put anyone off an ablation procedure as this is a matter between you and your medical team, but personally I wouldn't (and didn't!) rush to put a load of scar tissue in my heart when there were other things I could try first.

Having said this, I know of many people who have had very successful ablations and are now living happy lives a-fib free. My goal when writing this book was to share my story and help you achieve freedom from a-fib by whatever method works for you. If that is ablation no problem!

There are a few other treatments for a-fib which might be worth a mention, but they are not generally undertaken unless part of another procedure. The Maze Procedure, sometimes called the Cox-Maze method is a surgical procedure which is usually only done when the patient is having other heart surgery such as valve replacement. It involves making a maze pattern on the heart to stop the errant electrical signals travelling across the heart.

Most strokes from a-fib originate from blood clots which form in a part of the heart called the left atrial appendage. No-one knows what the left atrial appendage does, in that respect it is a lot like the appendix. However due to the shape of it (it is almost an ear shaped sac) it can form a pouch which can trap stagnant blood. If this blood clots and is then pumped out of the heart it could cause a stroke. For this reason, procedures to close off the left atrial appendage either by surgical means or by the implantation of a small umbrella device called the Watchman or a plug type device is available.

Closure of the left atrial appendage is sometimes recommended for patients who cannot take traditional blood thinners. Older style blood thinners such as Warfarin could be quite difficult to manage and required frequent testing of the patient to ensure levels weren't too high or too low. Too much anti-coagulation could lead to internal bleeding whereas not enough could lead to clots. The new generation of blood thinners are much easier for patients to tolerate, work just as effectively and don't require the intensive monitoring that Warfarin did.

WHY A-FIB IS OFTEN A DISEASE OF LIFESTYLE, NOT THE HEART

In the past few years, a-fib has become an epidemic. Once considered mainly a disease of elderly patients, more and more younger patients are developing a-fib. Just as diabetes is a ticking time bomb, a-fib has the potential to cripple the health service budget in the UK. So why is a-fib suddenly becoming such a big problem? Quite simply, as a nation we are becoming unhealthier.

If you were struck down with a-fib out of the blue, and you don't have any form of structural heart disease then it might be a sign that your body is crying out for help. Remember our Chinese friends who view a-fib as a symptom rather than a stand-alone disease?

Even in the most apparently healthy people, a-fib can be an indicator that all is not as well as it seems. Ironically, athletes particularly endurance athletes are very prone to a-fib. It is so well documented that marathon runners and cyclists are more likely than the average person to develop a-fib that some doctors routinely ask whether patients do either of these activities when faced with a young, apparently fit individual in the emergency

Jay Clarke

room.

When I was first diagnosed, I was a bit of a medical mystery. I wasn't too keen on being a medical mystery as it mainly seemed to involve troops of student doctors poking at me and umming and ahing at my bedside. For me, a-fib was a total bolt from the blue, I was young, active, no known health problems and never really had a day sick in my life.

Hindsight is an exact science but looking back I now realise I had been under a little more stress than usual in the lead up to my first episode, I wasn't eating particularly well and had generally not paid much attention to my health. I was busy living my life when wham, quite literally my heart felt like it was trying to escape from my body. My pulse was wild and erratic, and I could feel my heart pounding in my chest and an uncomfortable feeling in my throat. My heart continued its merry dance, bucking and whirling and I felt sick with terror. What on earth was going on? Was I about to die?

I tried lying down to see if it would calm down (luckily, I was at home and not in the street or office or someone would have undoubtedly called an ambulance or even an undertaker). It didn't calm down, but I didn't die either! After about fifteen minutes I decided I probably should seek some sort of medical attention, but I didn't think it warranted an ambulance, so I got a car up to the nearest emergency department. Typically, just before reaching the hospital I felt my heart calm down and the episode stopped as quickly as it began. By the time I was seen in the emergency department my heart was back in rhythm and an ECG showed absolutely nothing wrong.

Whether it was my insistence that I had just cheated death! or the fact they were having a quiet day in A & E, the doctor I saw did a complete work up and called down a cardiologist. Of course, my ECG was normal by now, but I was absolutely insistent that whatever I had experienced was not a panic attack. 'Describe what your pulse felt like during the episode' the cardiologist said. 'Beat the rhythm out on the table'. I did my best Keith Moon drumming impression. 'Ah' the cardiologist said. 'I think I know what just happened'.

For the next few days I became an unwilling participant in a series of medical experiments. I was x-rayed, given numerous ECGs and an echocardiogram for good measure, had copious amounts of blood removed, made to urinate in assorted containers, was probed by cold stethoscopes and even colder fingers, was peered at by medical students and finally given a completely clean bill of health. 'We think we know what the problem is' the consultant said. This was the first time I had ever even heard of atrial fibrillation and now the consultant was telling me I had it. 'The important thing to take is away is to know that this condition will not kill you' he went on. 'It is something you can live with for years and years and if it becomes a problem in the future, we can treat it'. And so, discharging me with a tightly sealed envelope to give to my doctor my journey with a-fib began.

Living With A-fib

Life with a-fib can be unpredictable and challenging. As I had paroxysmal a-fib there was no knowing when or where an attack would strike. There was no warning other than occasionally a few skipped beats in the minutes prior to an attack and episodes would stop as suddenly as they started.

Initially, I would have runs of just a few minutes, but they would soon start to extend into hours. Luckily my attacks never lasted more than a day, but I soon found myself frustrated, withdrawn and depressed. The doctor's advice of just live with it just wasn't working for me.

Questions directed at medical professions as to WHY this was happening to me went unanswered, my case went against everything they had every learned in medical school about a-fib. I was young, healthy, had no problems with my heart structurally or otherwise, no high blood pressure, I was moderately overweight with blood sugar slightly above normal but not in the diabetic range.

My thyroid (a potent trigger of a-fib) tested fine. I was declared a case of lone a-fib and told my stroke risk was so low I didn't warrant any form of anti-coagulants. If episodes lasted more than 48 hours I was to return to the emergency room for an attempt to convert my heart back into normal rhythm but thankfully that never happened as my events, although frequent always converted within 24 hours.

Back then much of the research into lifestyle factors and a-fib was in its infancy. At one point I was told that being overweight did not contribute to a-fib, but the LEGACY study later proved that was very much untrue. A-fib was treated purely as a cardiac condition or occasionally as a neurological condition and apart from the obvious diabetes and high blood pressure risk factors, not much notice was taken of the patients lifestyle.

I knew that if I was going to crack the mystery of why I was the 1 in 10,000 (figures from that period but now much higher) of my age-group who got a-fib I was going to have to figure it out for myself. This started me on a journey to learn everything I could about the condition, a journey which eventually led to my cure.

So What Really Causes A-fib?

In the absence of structural heart disease, I believe a-fib to be a symptom of a body out of balance. Now I know that sounds a bit vague and generalist but hear me out. There is no one reason fits all or magic bullet for this affliction. There are literally hundreds of reasons why your body goes into a-fib from the soda you drank in the morning to your high blood pressure putting extra strain on your heart.

The key is figuring out which of the causes of a-fib apply to you (and each person may have multiple risk factors) and taking steps to remedy each one to bring your body back in balance.

Strain on the body from any source, whether it be your insulin levels are too high or your diet is lacking essential vitamins and minerals causes inflammation within your body. Inflammation is the body's defence from attack, but it also can be very problematic, especially for the a-fib patient.

Levels of inflammation in the body can be tested by measuring a protein made by your liver called c-reactive protein. C-reactive protein is elevated when the body is under stress – and here's the kicker, people who have a-fib consistently have higher levels of c-reactive protein in their blood indicating a high level of inflammation.

(*C-reactive protein elevation in patients with atrial arrhythmias: inflammatory mechanisms and persistence of atrial fibrillation Chung et al.*)

So, we know that higher levels of inflammation in the body are associated with a-fib. We also know that raised levels of c-reactive protein can be used as a marker to predict future cardiovascular events. So, it stands to reason that if we reduce stress in the body and lower our c-reactive protein levels our inflammation levels will drop and so will our risk of cardiovascular events including a-fib.

Inflammation in your body will make it irritable. Our cranky atria are more likely to misbehave when there are high levels of inflammation as will our nervous system in general. The vagal nerve is one of the most important nerves in your body with multiple bodily functions coming under its control including the regulation of the heartbeat.

The vagal nerve alone when irritated can initiate an a-fib attack. These types of episodes usually begin in the evening or after a heavy meal and often resolve in the early hours. They are not associated with any form of heart disease and often happen in young, healthier people including marathon runners and athletes. They usually occur when relaxing or when the stomach is irritated by excess gas or being over full.

My own attacks can be classified as this type. They mostly occurred in the evening and for some reason often on Sundays, something I never did manage to figure out. My triggers were leaning forward, overeating, lying on my stomach, bending over and on one occasion shouting!

Anything that irritates or stimulates the vagal nerve can lead to an episode. But the vagal nerve is a lot more cranky when the body is under stress.

Before continuing, I thought I should explain more about what I mean by stress on the body. When we think of stress we tend to think of mental stress, pressures and worries. Whilst these can and do lead to inflammation, by stress I am referring to anything which interferes with the smooth running of the body.

There are literally thousands of things that cause stress on the body and cause it to become inflamed, far more than the scope of this book. However, I am going to discuss some of the most common factors that can contribute to a-fib that I discovered from my own research.

MAJOR STRESSORS TO THE HEART

If you are planning to have an a-fib attack, the holy trinity of ingredients would be high blood pressure, diabetes and obesity. All these factors on their own are more than enough to cause a-fib but when combined they are a deadly combination. The good thing is that every single one of them is a modifiable risk and can often be eliminated altogether.

High Blood Pressure

Firstly, high blood pressure. If you are planning to do just one thing to reduce your chances of going into a-fib and improving your cardiovascular health, it would be to get your blood pressure under control. Having blood pressure that is too high puts massive pressure on your cardiovascular system day in day out.

About 75% of people who have a stroke also have high blood pressure. So, you can reduce your stroke risk right off the bat by working to get your blood pressure under control.

Ideally your blood pressure should be between 90/60 and 120/80. Readings lower than 90/60 are classed as low and anything over 140/90 is high.

Luckily there are a lot of things you can do to reduce your blood pressure if it is high. Often doctors suggest lifestyle changes as a first line of attack before prescribing medication.

Five things you can do to lower your blood pressure

1. Exercise. Just being a little more active in your daily life can help to bring down your blood pressure. Walk for short journeys instead of taking the car, get up regularly and walk around instead of lazing in front of the TV and try to incorporate regular, gentle exercise into your daily routine. Start off slowly and always under the guidance of your doctor, particularly if you have other health issues.

2. Reduce your sodium intake. Salt encourages the body to hold on to fluid which in turn raises your blood pressure. Salt can also be a trigger for a-fib in itself. Avoid adding additional salt to your food and avoid cooking with it if you can. Processed foods are packed with salt.

3. Losing just 5% of your body weight could reduce your blood pressure significantly if you are overweight. Being overweight puts extra strain on your heart and even moderate weight loss is beneficial to your entire cardiovascular system.

4. Avoid alcohol. Alcohol can not only raise your blood pressure but it also bad for the heart in other ways too. Binge drinking is associated with episodes of a-fib even in people who have never had it before. This phenomenon is so common that doctors even have a name for it – 'holiday heart' as so many people are admitted to the ER during holidays due to excess alcohol. The UK guidelines suggest that men should consume no more than 3-4 units per day and women 2-3.

5. Eat foods rich in potassium. Potassium is an a-fib patients' friend as it helps the heart maintain a regular, steady rhythm. It also helps to reduce excess sodium which can excite the heart and helps to ease pressure on your blood vessels. And it can also help

to lower your blood pressure.

Normal potassium levels are between 3.6 and 5.2 millimoles per litre but many a-fib suffers have levels below 3.5 which is classed as low. In fact, if you have low potassium, getting it back into normal range may be all you need to do to say goodbye to a-fib forever.

Checking your potassium levels should be one of the first things doctors do when investigating a-fib but many patients have never had their levels checked and consequently could be walking around with dangerously low levels.

At one time, potassium deficiency was considered quite rare, but recently it has been proven to be a lot more widespread than previously thought. The recommended consumption of 3500mg to 4700mg a day is quite an ask for many people, especially if you are restricting calories or have a diet limited in fruit and vegetables.

Potassium supplements are not recommended as they can be quite dangerous unless taken under strict medical supervision. So much so that in most countries the maximum amount of potassium allowed in supplements is just 100mg, a fraction of the amount needed daily. Therefore, it is always best to ditch supplements (unless prescribed) and try and eat as many potassium rich foods as possible. Some potassium rich foods are listed under the section potassium further in this book.

A word of caution – if you have kidney disease you might need to restrict the amount of potassium in your diet. When kidneys aren't functioning effectively, they cannot clear excess potassium from the blood. It builds up and can be quite dangerous. One of the functions of dialysis is to try to remove excess potassium but you will be advised to limit foods rich in potassium between sessions.

Aim to get your blood pressure below 120/80 and ideally closer to 100/60 if you can.

Diabetes

High blood sugar disrupts just about every organ in the body, but it is especially damaging to the heart and cardiovascular system and the nervous system. This is why it often goes hand in hand with a-fib. The damage that years of chronically high blood sugar (even before it hits the diabetic range) can do is truly frightening, over 80% of diabetics die from either heart attack or stroke, not to mention the other horrific side effects such as blindness and loss of limbs. I am not trying to scare you, but if you, like me were complacent about the risks that higher than normal blood sugar brings, don't be. Do whatever you can to bring your blood sugar into the normal range. And the good news is, there is a lot you can do to help yourself.

For a long time, diabetes was considered a life-long, chronic and progressive condition, much the same as a-fib was. But we now know that diabetes is as reversible as a-fib for many people.

Our modern diet is loaded with refined carbs especially white flour and sugar. It is not a coincidence that the shift in diet from plant and meat-based foods towards "white carbs" such as bread, pasta and processed breakfast cereals has coincided with the rise in diabetes. Coupled with our more sedentary lifestyles, where we don't burn off the amount of carbs that our ancestors did, we now have a ticking health related time bomb. Over 10% of the US population now have diabetes and many more will be diagnosed in the coming years.

In the 1980's some health advice came out that unwittingly

helped to fuel the diabetes epidemic. We were told to eat low fat, high carb and that fat was the enemy that led to heart disease, obesity and a host of other horrible diseases. In the next couple of decades, we became fatter, more miserable and diabetic.

Whilst Dr Atkins did a good job of debunking the myth that fat is not the demon it is made out to be, it is only now that we are beginning to recognise the value of low carb, high fat diets in reversing many of the chronic diseases of our time, including diabetes, epilepsy and a-fib.

In order to understand why this is so relevant let's look at some of the thinking about diabetes and how it has changed over the last few years.

Firstly, though let's look at a very simplified model of how diabetes develops. When we eat food especially carbohydrate, our bodies convert it into glucose where it is broken down to produce energy which is used by our cells. The amount of glucose in our blood is controlled by the pancreas which produces insulin. The job of insulin is to transport the glucose out of our blood stream and into our cells.

However, when insulin doesn't work properly, either because there is not enough of it or more likely the cells become resistant to it we have a problem. The glucose stays in our blood stream and blood sugar levels begin to rise. Eventually, diabetes develops.

Firstly though, the body attempts to compensate by producing more and more insulin. Now insulin is known as the fat-storing hormone so as insulin levels rise it becomes easier and easier to store fat. Not only do we become fatter, but we are also well on the road to diabetes. The body cells become more resistant to the ever-rising insulin levels and our blood sugar starts to get higher and higher. Ironically, we often give diabetics who already have extremely high insulin levels, even more insulin and wonder why they gain weight or feel even sicker.

At this point, I need to make it clear I am only talking about Type 2 diabetes which makes up around 90% of diabetes diagnoses. Type 1 diabetes is a completely different condition where the pancreas doesn't produce enough insulin to control the blood sugar levels. Type 1 diabetics need to take insulin every day whereas initially Type 2 diabetes is often controlled by diet and exercise.

Now this is where old and modern thinking collide. In the old days, diabetes was considered a disease of a 'worn-out' pancreas, it was thought that once the beta cells in the pancreas which produce insulin no longer worked effectively, that was that and the patient was diabetic for life.

BUT

In the UK, a diabetes research team at Newcastle University, led by Professor Roy Taylor had come up with a very different hypothesis. Professor Taylor believed that diabetes wasn't caused by a worn-out pancreas at all, but by a fatty liver, a condition that many of us live with but don't even know it. He believed that by unclogging the liver and pancreas by the use of a very strict medically supervised 800 calorie a day diet for a short period, the patients' blood sugar levels would return to normal.

By shedding fat around the liver and pancreas, the participants in the Newcastle study did indeed achieve remission from diabetes. Initial results showed that just under 50% who successfully completed the diet were diabetes free 12 months later.

Since then, other studies have proved Professor Taylors hypothesis to be true and now diabetes is considered in many cases to be a reversible condition. In fact, it was proved that it wasn't necessary to undergo the 800 calorie a day diet and that any weight loss combined with restriction of carbohydrates would work effectively.

Restricting carbohydrates however is essential to give the pancreas a rest whilst allowing the liver and pancreas time to unclog. If you continue to bombard your cells with a huge supply of glucose, they will never have the time to recover function effectively.

The body can store around 48-72 hours' worth of glucose in the liver in the form of glycogen. When you restrict carbohydrates, the body first uses the glycogen stored in the liver to fuel the body's essential processes. When that supply runs out, the body must turn to fat for fuel. This is a process known as ketosis and it usually starts 2-3 days after carbohydrate restriction. Ketosis or keto as it is often known burns the body's own fat for fuel which is why it is such an effectively weight loss method.

Once the body is effectively in ketosis, most people report that they have never felt better, they feel energised and full of life. The first few days can be a little rough and it is very important to maintain hydration whilst on a ketogenic diet to avoid some of the most common initial problems such as headache and fatigue.

You can read lots about ketogenic diets and how they could reverse diabetes online, just about every diabetic forum has success stories from people who have achieved normal blood sugar levels, some in just a few days.

A word of warning, if you are thinking of changing your way of eating, particularly if you are on medication or insulin then it is really important to do this only with the express permission and monitoring of your health care provider. Ketogenic diets can be very effective, they will drop your blood sugar massively in just a few days so your medication needs to be carefully monitored and reduced if necessary.

So, what can you eat on a ketogenic diet?

Lean meat, fish, eggs, cheese, most fats, some veggies such as leafy green vegetables, some fruits and berries and certain nuts including pecans, brazil nuts and almonds.

Avoid bread, baked goods, potatoes (small amounts of sweet potato are ok on some plans), rice, pasta, sugar, anything made with flour, cereals.

The Atkins diet suggests reducing carbohydrates to under 20g a day for the first 14 days but for most people this is very restrictive and unsustainable. 50g of carbs per day is perhaps more achievable but still quite restrictive whereas others aim for 75g-100g of carbs per day which is about half to a third of the amount of carbs most people consume every day.

If you are used to the modern American/British diet you will find it quite tough going for the first few days. The thing with keto is unlike other diets, if you cheat and splurge on carbs you will set yourself back 2-3 days while your body goes back into ketosis.

Why Diabetes Makes A-Fib Worse.

High blood sugar causes inflammation in the body. A-fib sufferers are known to have higher than normal markers of inflammation in their blood anyway but coupled with diabetes it is a double whammy. Inflammation directly affects the myocardium of the heart and the autonomic nervous system making it much more likely to initiate an episode of a-fib.

So, one of the first goals in reversing your a-fib must be to get your blood sugar under control. Even before levels hit the marker for a diagnosis of diabetes, the irritation to the heart that increased glucose and high levels of insulin cause make you much more susceptible to a-fib.

You can buy cheap glucose monitors at any pharmacy or your doctor can give you a simple finger prick test which will instantly give you a reading of your blood sugar levels. A better test is the hbA1c test which gives an average read of your blood sugar levels over the past 2-3 months.

The US uses the mg/dL system to measure blood sugar levels whereas the UK uses mmol/L. It doesn't really matter which system you measure in as the results are the same. An ideal fasting blood sugar level is less than 100mg/dL or 5.6 mmol/L. Levels between 100 to 125 mg/dL (5.6 to 6.9 mmol/L) indicate prediabetes whereas levels over 126 mg/dL (7 mmol/L) measured on two separate occasions are indicative of diabetes. Fasting blood sugar is measured after a period of 8 hours without food.

Obesity

The third factor which increases your risk of a-fib is obesity. In fact, recently, it has been shown that obesity is even higher a risk factor for a-fib than previously thought. **One in five cases of a-fib are now believed to be attributable to obesity alone**. The good news? Weight-loss can reduce and even cure a-fib altogether. So, if there is ever a reason to try to shed those excess pounds this is it.

An Australian study at the University of Adelaide found that just a 10% drop in bodyweight could reverse a-fib. 88% of the 355 patients studied who managed to lose 10% of their starting bodyweight became either a-fib free or had their episodes reduce from persistent to paroxysmal.

So why does obesity go hand in hand with a-fib? Excess weight remodels the atria – rather like blowing up a balloon they get bigger and begin to stretch. This stretch interrupts the normal electrical systems making a-fib much more likely to occur. Weight loss can reverse this condition, bringing the atria down to more normal size and structure.

Not only that, remember our old friend c-reactive protein? That annoying marker of inflammation in our bodies? Well obesity causes inflammation, lots of it. And we know that inflammation causes a-fib. So, the more weight you gain, the more your c-reactive protein levels rise. Your body comes under stress and not surprisingly, the electrical system in your heart starts to act out too.

Weight loss and gentle exercise can help to reverse the levels of inflammation in your body as well as being beneficial to just about every part of your health. Weight loss can help to reduce blood pressure as well as improving blood sugar and your overall cardiovascular health, it reduces the stress and strain on your bones, it improves your self-esteem and your mood and even helps you to think more clearly. Your energy levels will rise and even the most modest of weight loss can bring a massive improvement in the way you feel.

Studies have linked weight loss with a six-fold increase in arrythmia free survival. If that isn't enough motivation here's another statistic. In the Adelaide study 45% of participants who lost 10% of their body weight and kept their weight stable for four years were completely free of a-fib symptoms, without surgery or medications!

Whilst thin people do get a-fib (because there are a thousand reasons why a-fib develops) being overweight is a huge risk factor and one which is relatively easy to tackle. The key to reversing your a-fib with weight loss is gentle and sustained effort, fad diets might make the inflammation in your body worse. One thing the Adelaide study did find was that the weight loss needs to be sustained for the best results. If your weight fluctuates by more than

5% of your body weight, then you will not have as much success in reversing your a-fib as someone whose weight doesn't fluctuate. Therefore, aim to lose weight slowly and gently and try to keep it off.

I had been on diets in the past, but in the time before my diagnosis my weight had crept higher and higher. I had packed on the pounds due to a diet of junk food, a lack of exercise and a general apathy towards doing anything constructive about my weight. Indeed, at the time of diagnosis I was told that my weight had nothing to do with my condition, something which I now realise to be very untrue!

Lastly one often overlooked factor is that if you do go down the route of having an ablation, patients who are overweight have worse success rates than those who are of normal weight. Losing weight however might just prevent your need for an ablation anyway!

YOUR INITIAL ACTION PLAN TO TACKLE A-FIB

I am going to place a bet with you. I am willing to bet that if you tackle the critical 3 factors in beating a-fib – blood pressure, blood sugar and weight that your condition and cardiovascular health will improve significantly. Inflammation in your body will start to reduce, you will feel healthier and happier, and that might be all that is needed to wave goodbye to a-fib forever.

So, the very first thing you need to do is know your numbers. Get your blood pressure checked, your blood sugar levels and an accurate reading of your weight, preferable one with a body fat analysis. Fat is hyper-inflammatory so as you see your body fat percentage start to reduce you will know that you are starting to reduce your inflammation levels as well as looking and feeling better.

So your first challenge.
1. Aim to get your blood pressure to a reading of 120/80 preferable closer to 100/60 if you can manage it. Blood pressure varies throughout the day so if you can take several readings at different times to ensure you are getting an accurate picture. Your doctor might be able to help with ambulatory monitoring which is a 24 hour or longer reading of your blood pressure as you go about your daily tasks. But so long as you know your average numbers

and are working at getting them to a healthy level you will be doing the best thing you can to help your heart and reverse your a-fib.

2. Aim for normal blood sugar levels. Even slightly raised blood sugar levels are pro-inflammatory, and this happens way before the cut-off point for a diagnosis of diabetes. Restricting carbs is probably the easiest and fastest way to get your blood sugar down quickly but speak to your doctor before changing your diet, especially if you are on medication.

3.Lose weight if you are overweight. As we have seen backed up by solid medical research, your weight does matter when it comes to a-fib. Losing 10% of your body weight if you are overweight can cause you to lose a-fib altogether. The more obese you are, the more effective these measures are likely to be. The heart has an amazing ability to remodel itself when weight is lost, reducing atrial stretch, overall size and repairing the electrical system.

Keeping the weight off is crucial to long term success in reversing a-fib. Remember those in the study who lost the weight and kept it off remained a-fib free whereas those who yoyo-ed and gained and lost more than 5% of their body weight had many more symptoms. And if you are in the 20% of people whose a-fib is solely down to their weight then you are likely to get rid of a-fib altogether!

THE VAGAL NERVE
AND A-FIB

The vagal (vagus) nerve is the longest nerve in the human body. Its job is to provide and control the parasympathetic (calming) response to the major organs, including the heart, lungs and digestive tract. If your heart acts up and skips beats when you have eaten or you feel gassy, the chances are that the vagal nerve is the culprit.

Lots of things can cause the vagal nerve to misfire, including gas or a full stomach pressing on your diaphragm, being overweight, leaning forward, being under stress, having a vitamin or mineral deficiency or even just relaxing at the end of the day! But when the vagal nerve is irritable it can send errant signals to the atria which result in an a-fib attack.

At one time, a-fib was divided into two 'varieties' – adrenergic and vagal depending on the characteristics of each episode. This classification system has fallen out of use with time but for this chapter it might be useful to go back and revisit it.

The autonomic nervous system (also known as the unconscious or involuntary nervous system) regulates bodily functions such as your heart rate, breathing, digestion, body temperature and all of the processes which occur "automatically" in your body. It can be divided into three parts, the sympathetic nervous system which controls your fight or flight response, the parasympathetic nervous system which controls your bodies response during rest and relaxation and the enteric nervous system which controls digestion and your gut.

To simplify things somewhat imagine a car. Step on the gas and pull away, that's your sympathetic nervous system working. When you press on the brake and start to slow down, that's your parasympathetic nervous system taking control.

So, what has all this got to do with a-fib? Going back to the two 'varieties' of a-fib, adrenergic a-fib is triggered by the sympathetic nervous system whereas vagal a-fib is triggered by the parasympathetic nervous system – that pesky vagal nerve again.

Adrenergic a-fib occurs when the body is under stress, whether from a flood of adrenaline (the fight or flight response), or exercise, exertion, stimulants or a perceived threat. It usually occurs mainly in the daytime and is more likely to be associated with structural heart disease than vagal a-fib.

On the other hand, vagal a-fib tends to occur when the body is resting or digesting a meal. It often comes on in the evenings and converts in the early morning hours. This type of a-fib is seldom associated with structural heart disease and stems instead from an imbalance in the nervous system, an irritable vagal nerve. Bending, coughing, stretching, even straining on the toilet can bring on this type of a-fib but from a positive point of view, this is a type of a-fib that rarely progresses to permanent.

If you have gastric problems as well as a-fib, the two are most likely linked by an issue with your vagal nerve. If your a-fib comes on when you are relaxing in the evening or after eating a heavy meal that is another clue that the vagal nerve is the culprit.

So, what causes the vagal nerve or indeed any part of the nervous system to act up? In short, a body out of balance, one that is strug-

Jay Clarke

gling with high levels of inflammation.

To get your nervous system back into shape, create a plan to reduce the inflammation in your body. If you want to monitor how you are doing, get a blood test to measure your levels of c-reactive protein. An ideal level is less than 1. Anything higher suggests that you have a problem with inflammation.

Things That Cause Inflammation.

1. A high sugar junk food diet. A diet which is packed with processed food and empty calories, not only depletes your body of vitamins and minerals, it also causes chronic inflammation.

2. A lack of exercise. As little as 20 minutes of exercise has been found to have significant anti-inflammatory effects on the body.

3, Inflammatory fats such as processed vegetable oils and trans fats. Switch to heart healthy fats such as olive oil and choose oily fish such as tuna and mackerel for their Omega 3 content.

4. Stress – mental stress increases inflammation so try to actively relax. Switch off screens, go for a walk, try meditation or even take up yoga. Yoga has been found to have a beneficial effect on a-fib by shortening episodes as well as decreasing stress and inflammation.

5. Keep your blood sugar in normal range. High blood sugar has a pro-inflammatory effect on the body so aim to keep it under control.

6. Vitamin and mineral deficiencies. Anything the body needs but lacks will cause an increase in inflammation. Real food is the best way to nourish your body, but a multivitamin may help to ad-

dress a deficiency in the short term. One study found that a daily good quality multivitamin could help lower c-reactive protein levels.

7. Food intolerances and sensitivities. Whilst gluten, soy and dairy are some of the more common food intolerances, anything that your body perceives to be a threat will trigger inflammation. Try keeping a food diary and experiment by removing foods that you think may be causing a problem.

RULE OUT SLEEP APNEA

The link between sleep apnea and a-fib has been recognised for many years, yet it is a condition which often goes undiagnosed. Sleep apnea alone can be the cause of a-fib and simply treating the condition may be enough to make your a-fib go away altogether. If you snore, particularly if it is loud enough to keep other bed or housemates awake at night, consider getting a sleep study done.

Obstructive sleep apnea causes you to stop breathing many times per night. You might not even remember these episodes in the morning although you might suffer from daytime drowsiness and irritability. One study found that around 40% of people who have a-fib also have sleep apnea, and yet another one estimated the true number to be at least 80%. It also works the other way, if you have a-fib but no sleep apnea, your chances of developing it are more than 4 times that of those without a-fib.

Sleep apnea can remodel the heart in the same way as untreated a-fib. It is known that as your body weight increases, so does your chance of developing sleep apnea.

Likewise, as you lose weight sleep apnea improves and often disappears altogether. Sleep apnea alone can cause weight gain and when the condition is controlled, it often becomes much easier to lose weight.

A sleep study is used to diagnose sleep apnea and this is carried out in a special clinic or at home. Depending on the degree of sleep interruption, it is classified as either none, mild, moderate or severe. If you are on the milder end of the spectrum, lifestyle measures such as losing weight or stopping smoking might be all that is needed.

Moderate to severe apnea is treated using a CPAP machine. This machine has a mask which is worn at night which uses mild air pressure to hold the airway open.

When untreated, sleep apnea can be a serious condition with some nasty side effects, a-fib being just one of them. In the very worst case scenario, it could cause a rare type of right sided heart failure called cor pulmonale. This is why it is important to recognise and treat it in the a-fib patient.

MAGNESIUM – THE MIRACLE MINERAL?

Did you know that over 80% of the population are deficient in magnesium? Magnesium is a mineral that is crucial to a healthy heartbeat, yet 4/5ths of us are severely lacking. If you have a-fib, diabetes, metabolic syndrome, or raised blood sugar, you are almost certainly deficient in this miracle mineral.

Magnesium is responsible for over 300 functions in the human body, yet the amount we get from our diets has been declining rapidly for many years. Between 1940 and 1991, the magnesium levels in vegetables dropped by 24% and in fruit by 16% due to mineral depletion in soil.

A-fib has been cited as a symptom of magnesium deficiency and that even a short-term deficiency could provoke a-fib in even healthy people with no known arrythmia. In 2007 an interesting study proved this assumption to be right, albeit with a small sample of participants.

The study set out to find whether even a short-term mineral deficiency could provoke arrythmias in post-menopausal women. The researchers cut the magnesium in the diet of the test subjects to just one third of the RDA for just over two months and would then replace the missing magnesium for a further period of 58 days.

What happened was that nearly a third of the participants had to enter the replacement phase early due to the heart rhythm changes that occurred. Nearly a quarter of the participants developed a-fib or a-flutter despite never having had the arrythmia before. If ever there was an indicator that even short-term magnesium deficiency could provoke a-fib it was this study.

And many of us are chronically deficient in this essential mineral.

Only about 1% of the magnesium contained in the body is present in the blood, so standard blood tests are not that good at diagnosing a deficiency. And to add to the problem, it can take a long time to correct even a small deficiency!

Symptoms of a Magnesium Deficiency

Muscle twitching, spasms, tics
Irritability
Anxiety and panic attacks
Tiredness and lethargy
Inability to sleep
Inability to "Switch Off"
Seizures
Irregular or rapid heartbeat
Coronary spasms
Potassium deficiency
Impaired glucose tolerance
Hyperglycaemia
Tremors

Difficulty swallowing
Dizziness
Numbness and tingling
PMS
High blood pressure
Carb cravings
Craving for salt
Insomnia
Loss of appetite
Nausea
GERD
Confusion
Personality changes
Asthma and breathing difficulties
Chronic fatigue syndrome
ADHD
Tooth decay
Gum disease.

Why Magnesium is a great anti-arrhythmic

Magnesium plays an important role in the electrical function of the heart. Together with potassium and sodium it helps keep the heart beat stable and steady. Magnesium prolongs the atrial and atrioventricular rest period and slows conduction times. Atrial tissue with inadequate magnesium is electrically unstable and irritable.

How To Correct A Magnesium Deficiency

A magnesium deficiency can take a long time to correct. Magnesium supplementation is generally considered very safe in people with normal kidney function but as with everything please check with your doctor before taking any sort of supplement.

Magnesium needs a sufficient supply of potassium in your body in order to absorb optimally so if your potassium is low you might need to fix this before your magnesium levels will rise. Potassium supplementation is very much a matter for your doctors' supervision as potassium can be dangerous if taken incorrectly.

Another problem with correcting a magnesium deficiency is that the lower your levels are, the less your body will absorb!

To raise your magnesium levels naturally, try to incorporate as many magnesium rich foods into your diet as possible. Good dietary sources of magnesium are:

Pumpkin Seeds
Spinach
Swiss Chard
Yoghurt/Kefir
Almonds
Black Beans
Avocado
Figs
Dark Chocolate
Banana
Salmon
Nuts and Seeds
Coriander
Coffee Kelp
Rice Bran

Magnesium Supplementation

If you choose to take a magnesium supplement, some forms of magnesium are much better absorbed than others. Magnesium oxide is the most easily found form of magnesium supplement but unfortunately it is not well absorbed at all. Only around 4% of the magnesium oxide in a standard 500mg tablet is available to the body.

More absorbable forms of magnesium are magnesium glycinate, magnesium taurate and magnesium citrate. Magnesium glycinate is less likely to cause loose stools than other forms of magnesium and has the highest bioavailability with about 80% of each dose being absorbed.

Magnesium taurate is a compound of magnesium and taurine which is an amino acid. Taurine dampens the activity of the sympathetic nervous system so may be useful for adrenally driven forms of a-fib.

Magnesium citrate is cheap and easy to find, as well as being relatively well absorbed. Unfortunately, it does have a downside and that is the laxative effects it causes at higher doses. It is also excreted quite quickly by the body so if you choose this type of magnesium, experiment with a dose that doesn't cause you bowel problems and then split the dose over the course of a day.

Another form of magnesium, and one which comes without the laxative effect of oral forms is transdermal magnesium. This is a topical form of magnesium chloride which is often used by sportspeople for treating aches, pains and injuries.

Transdermal magnesium is sometimes called magnesium oil, although it is not really an oil at all. The best quality versions are made from a 31% solution of magnesium chloride dissolved in purified water.

Transdermal magnesium can replete magnesium stores approximately 5 times faster than oral magnesium supplements and has none of the laxative side effects. Use it on unbroken skin (note it might sting a little on first application particularly if you are very low in magnesium). On average you will see results after about 6 weeks of transdermal magnesium use, whereas it can take 6 months or longer for oral magnesium supplements to work.

Epsom salts are another type of magnesium, but they are not recommended for use as a magnesium supplement. For one, they have a very potent laxative effect and secondly, they are much less effective than other forms of magnesium. They are still used primarily in bath salts and they might raise magnesium levels very slightly but not enough to make a significant difference.

Magnesium Overdose

Magnesium is generally considered very safe and effective when used in the proper manner but although rare, magnesium overdose can occur. This usually only happens in people with kidney problems or when very large amounts of magnesium are ingested. Nevertheless, get medical advice before taking any type of supplement to be on the safe side.

Signs of Magnesium Overdose
Low blood pressure
Slow breathing
Slow heart rate and or erratic heart rhythm
Shortness of breath
Dizziness
In very severe cases cardiac arrest

Seek immediate medical attention if you suspect a magnesium overdose.

DIET – COULD MY DIET BE CONTRIBUTING TO A-FIB?

Your body is essentially an engine which needs high quality fuel to keep it functioning optimally. Unfortunately, the modern diet which is high in processing and often low in nutrients does not always provide the best fuel for your engine.

Vitamin and mineral deficiencies and food intolerances/allergies stress your engine even more. Sugar depletes just about every vitamin and mineral but especially magnesium which is crucial for maintaining a healthy heartbeat and nervous system.

If you eat foods which you know cause you problems, you will increase the inflammatory response in your body and make your atria even more cranky.

I am the worlds biggest fan of junk food, I love bread, pasta, anything sweet and I can eat ice cream by the gallon. I consistently over-fuelled my body with junk and then I acted surprised when my engine started to misfire. I won't pretend that I completely overhauled my diet, I am still likely to try to fight you for the last cookie in the jar!

But what I did was try to increase my intake of healthy, unprocessed foods and paid attention to the vitamin and mineral content of what I was eating to ensure that I did at least come up to the RDA in what I needed. Then, when I did indulge I could do so without guilt.

During my research, I found that some food stuffs, in particular certain food additives came up time and time again when people listed their triggers for a-fib. Here's what I discovered.

MSG – Monosodium Glutamate, Vetsin or E621

MSG is a controversial subject, the latest research says that there is no link between MSG and atrial fibrillation, yet many a-fibbers reports a sensitivity to this commonly used additive, myself included.

MSG is a flavour enhancer and it appears in a ton of savoury and processed products, especial Asian cuisine, ready meals, snack foods and sauces and dressings. MSG sensitivity was once dubbed "Chinese Restaurant syndrome" as so many people reported a reaction to Asian food which contained MSG. These days many restaurants choose to cook without it, but it can still be found in abundance in savoury, processed foods.

The science behind MSG causing issues is actually quite solid. MSG competes in the body for cysteine, which is needed by the body to create taurine, an amino acid which is essential for maintaining a regular, steady heartbeat.

Symptoms of MSG intolerance usually start within a couple of hours of consuming food containing MSG and include an irregular or erratic heartbeat, racing heart, premature contractions of the heart which can be perceived as 'skipped beats', headache, flushing, nausea and sweating, numbness and a feeling of burning in the mouth.

A doctor who personally suffered from a-fib tried an experiment. He cut out all foods containing MSG and aspartame from his diet and his episodes stopped altogether. To test whether it was the MSG and aspartame that had really been triggering his episodes he set himself a challenge. He deliberately ate foods containing MSG or aspartame to see if he went back into a-fib. He did. So, there is some very compelling evidence that MSG is a trigger for some people.

It is my opinion that MSG serves to irritate an already cranky nervous system and thus can contribute to a-fib in this way. I myself have had problems with MSG but I noticed that when I started to raise my magnesium levels (thus calming the nervous system) MSG did not affect me quite so badly.

Aspartame

Aspartame is another ingredient that seems to be able to provoke arrythmias in vulnerable hearts. Its use as an artificial sweetener (additive E951) means it is found abundantly in our low calorie, diet conscious society. It is commonly used in diet drinks such as soda, low calorie sweeteners, desserts and even some places you wouldn't expect to find it such as toothpaste and vitamins.

Most people, even a-fibbers don't have problems with aspartame but I have included it as a few certainly do.

Wine, Cheese, Chocolate and Salami

What do the above all have in common, apart from tasting nice of course? They are all high in a substance called tyramine which can trigger arrythmias in some people. Tyramine occurs naturally in certain foods particularly aged and fermented cheeses, red wine, dark chocolate, smoked meats, bananas and even yoghurt.

If you notice your a-fib getting worse after eating any of these foods, tyramine could be the culprit.

Alcohol

A-fib can be a consequence of binge drinking even in people who have never suffered from a-fib before. It is well known that during holidays or other times when people overindulge in alcohol, hospital admissions for a-fib soar. Once the alcohol has left the system, the heart usually returns to normal and that is the end of the matter. This scenario is so familiar to emergency room staff that it has been given a name – holiday heart.

Why alcohol causes a-fib has been a matter for much debate although no-one doubts that it does. Alcohol dehydrates the body, can stimulate adrenaline release and depletes essential vitamins and minerals such as magnesium and potassium.

Whilst alcohol in excess can lead to a-fib what about light or moderate drinking? Here, the jury is still out. Some people seem to be very sensitive to alcohol whereas others can tolerate large amounts without issue. Red wine and certain spirits seem more likely to initial an episode than a couple of beers.

Shortly after being first diagnosed I found that I couldn't tolerate alcohol at all. Even one drink would lead to a racing heart and an uncomfortable feeling. Ironic as previously I had been quite a party animal in my youth.

However, I found as I improved my nutrition and especially worked on optimising my magnesium and minerals, I began to tolerate alcohol much better. This fits with my hypothesis that my nervous system was super-sensitive from being deprived of essential minerals for so long.

Food Sensitivities/Allergies and Intolerances

Anything which the body perceives as a threat will increase inflammation. For some people that may be wheat or gluten, for others it is dairy, and some have a serious allergy to nuts. The different between a food allergy and a food intolerance is that an allergy provokes an immune response, whereas an intolerance brings on symptoms which may vary with the length and type of exposure. The result is a stress on the body, and we know that stress causes inflammation which might provoke a-fib.

If you suspect that you have a food intolerance it is worth keeping a food diary and write down any symptoms you have after eating certain foods. Food allergies are more serious and can even be life threatening, so professional testing and proper medical advice is essential.

Gluten sensitivity is known to be a particular problem for some a-fib patients, and those suffering from coeliac disease seem to be more prone to a-fib than the general population. Dramatic improvements in a-fib has been seen by some people adopting a gluten free diet so if you think you may have a sensitivity to wheat or gluten, this may be a sensible starting point.

Caffeine

The latest research shows no link between a-fib and moderate caffeine consumption as was previously thought. Caffeine can however raise your blood pressure and your heart rate temporarily so if you already suffer from high blood pressure you might want to exercise some caution. However, for most people, moderate caffeine consumption will not impact their a-fib.

OTHER THINGS THAT MAY CONTRIBUTE TO A-FIB

I have tried to cover most of the major factors which can contribute to a-fib, but here are a few more things which you may not have considered.

Thyroid

Both an under and an overactive thyroid can contribute to a-fib, but an overactive thyroid is most often associated with the condition. The link between thyroid and a-fib is so well known that most hospital admissions for a first-time episode will include a thyroid test as standard. However, sometimes this is missed so if you haven't been tested recently it may be worthwhile getting checked. Correcting your thyroxine level may be all that is needed to make a-fib go away.

H Pylori

H-pylori is a bug that lives in the stomachs of many people. For most people it doesn't cause a problem but for others, it can cause ulcers and stomach issues. It is also linked to a-fib as it can cause inflammation in the gut.

If you have ever had a stomach ulcer, or if you have ongoing gastric issues along with your a-fib, it is worth getting checked for this little critter. It can be detected in blood, stool or breath samples and can be treated with a triple dose of antibiotics and acid reducing drugs.

Potassium Levels

Low potassium levels are associated with all sorts of arrythmias including very dangerous ones. If you haven't already, get your potassium checked and follow medical advice to ensure your potassium levels are adequate.

Don't take potassium supplements without the advice of the doctor, excessive potassium is as dangerous as low levels. For this reason, over the counter supplements are limited to 99mg of potassium. Correcting a potassium deficiency needs intensive monitoring by a medical professional.

Mercury fillings/Oral Health

Mercury does produce low levels of electrical current in the mouth and it has been suggested that this might contribute to a-fib. For this reason, some patients have gone down the route of having all their mercury fillings removed and replaced.

Personally, I don't think this is necessary, and as well as being expensive if not done meticulously could lead to the release of even more mercury.

However, I do believe that good oral health is critical to the a-fib patient. It has been known for a long time that gum disease increases the risk of cardiovascular problems, but a recent study also linked periodontal disease to the development of a-fib.

Extreme Exercise

Lone a-fib has long been associated with endurance athletes such as marathon runners, cyclists and swimmers. Endurance sports put the body under stress and can lead to dehydration and depletion of essential minerals such as magnesium and potassium. This in turn can trigger a-fib even in the most athletic of hearts.

HOW I CURED MY A-FIB. MY JOURNEY.

This is the way the world ends
Not with a bang but a whimper. TS Eliot

I think the above quote from TS Eliot sums up the end of my journey with a-fib. If you are expecting me to say I did one thing and I was suddenly cured, I am sorry to disappoint you. I would love to tell you that there is one easy step, one simple thing to do which will guarantee you will never have another episode again. But I am no charlatan, and this is an honest account of my journey with an unfathomable disease. A-fib has many causes and many cures.

I cannot tell you the single thing I did that led to my cure, but I can tell you that is was the cumulative effect of the things I tried that gave me freedom. From my years of research, I have found that the only way to view a-fib is from a holistic viewpoint and not as a standalone disease. In the absence of structural heart disease, a-fib is a symptom of imbalance in the body. The key is figuring out where that imbalance lies and correcting it.

I spent a long time floundering around, trying to find that one thing that would make that magic difference. Then one day during a thunderstorm the following thought occurred to me. For lightning to happen the conditions must be right. There must be an imbalance between storm clouds themselves or storm clouds and the ground. And for a-fib to occur there has to be an imbalance in the electrical system of the heart. In the absence of structural a-fib where the heart itself creates the imbalance, there must be something else going on elsewhere.

I suspect that the most crucial things I did overall was lose weight, change my diet and correct my nutritional deficiencies. In turn, that would have reduced my levels of c-reactive protein (I really wish I had the figures from my diagnosis so I could prove that is indeed the case) and calmed my vagal nerve which seemed to be the source of so much of my trouble.

Firstly though, I was thrown a curve ball. I ignored my weight for a long time as I had been told that it had no effect on a-fib whatsoever, thinking we now know to be completely flawed. In fact, my weight increased and my episodes increased and I still did not make the connection!

For a long time I believed that magnesium was the answer to curing my a-fib and whilst it helped significantly it did not completely eliminate my episodes. What it did do, is reduce the amount of PAC's I had (premature beats coming from the atria) which often precede or even induce an episode of a-fib. My heart felt calmer and |I felt calmer. My episodes got shorter in duration and I found I might even be able to stop an episode altogether with my go-to cure – orange juice and a couple of magnesium citrate tablets. I most certainly did have a long-standing magnesium deficiency which did not help the situation. I was prone to panic attacks which are a symptom of magnesium deficiency and on a checklist of deficiency symptoms I could check off virtually every one.

As I have mentioned, magnesium deficiency is epidemic in the modern population. If you have high blood sugar, you almost certainly have a deficiency. It's something which is difficult to diagnose as only 1% of the body's magnesium is present in the blood. So, you can have a massive deficiency without ever testing deficient on a blood test.

I have read many stories of people having a lot of success with magnesium alone, it has eliminated a-fib altogether in some people. So, it always worth giving it a try so long as you use on of the bio-available forms of magnesium I mentioned earlier and use it long enough to make a difference. A couple of magnesium oxide tablets just won't cut it.

So I had made good strides in eliminating my a-fib, my episodes were much shorter and further apart. During this period, I actually went a full year without an a-fib episode which from daily attacks was an amazing improvement. Then, shortly after Christmas (a time of great stress and overindulgence for many of us) wham I went into a-fib for one of the longest episodes I had ever had. In hindsight, I had created the perfect storm for my vagal nerve. I had overindulged, eaten way too much food, been under a lot of stress to create the perfect family Christmas and of course more than a few drops of alcohol had passed by my lips.

At the time though, I was pretty dispirited. I went to see my doctor who recommended an ablation. No, I am going to do this on my own I said, pig-headed as ever. He rolled his eyes and let me get on with it.

Next I looked at my diet. Keeping a food diary was a shocking record of exactly how bad the food choices I made were. No wonder my nervous system was so cranky when it was habitually fed on a diet of sugar, white carbs and other nutritionally empty calories.

My blood sugar had been diagnosed as borderline high, so I needed to get that down into a healthy range. This is where I made a bad decision.

I decided to go on a VLCD – a very low-calorie diet – the same type of diet that the Newcastle Researchers would later use to reverse diabetes. Unfortunately, the diet I chose was not a medically supervised diet like the Newcastle study and wasn't recommended for anyone with health problems. Living on 600 calories a day is no fun anyway, and after just two weeks I started to have the most horrendous palpitations. Now I am no stranger to palpitations as is anyone with a-fib but these were stronger and more sinister feeling. This is why I would never recommend such a diet to anyone, if you must do a VLCD make sure it is a medically approved and supervised one.

I had to come off the diet as I was genuinely convinced I was about to go into an even more sinister rhythm than a-fib but at the same time something interesting had happened. My blood sugar had dropped down to normal and I was also 10lbs lighter. And when I came off the diet and went back to eating normal food, my blood sugar stayed in the normal range. My weight however crept back up. I now know that a lot of that 10lbs I had lost suddenly was water weight and when I went back to eating normally it was inevitable that I would put several pounds back on.

This is when I learned about the keto diet. I had read the Dr Atkins diet book many years previously, but it had all been a bit too extreme for me, although the science behind it made sense. Most of all I was lured by the promise of never being hungry, as I was the sort of person who could happily nibble for every waking hour and still wake up in the night starving hungry. Now I know I can blame that squarely on my insulin levels which were making me ravenous

I adapted relatively easily to the keto diet, even as dyed in the wool carb lover I found plenty of things that I could eat. But what I found the most motivating about the keto diet was that I was no longer hungry. For someone who had previously got up in the night looking for something to snack on, this was truly life changing.

Although keto worked for me, I don't think that it was the method I chose to lose weight but the weight loss itself that made the difference. I truly believe that any diet which leads to sustained weight loss would have the same effect. And I did feel a difference, almost immediately the weight started to come off.

Prior to attempting to fix my nutritional deficiencies and losing weight, my a-fib had been very violent, I could feel every episode and every skipped beat, my heart would hammer and leap around for hours as if a crazy out of step marching band was attempting to burst through my chest. How I envied those who didn't feel their a-fib.

The magnesium had calmed my heart down a lot, it had shortened the episodes and made them less violent. But, shortly after starting to lose weight in earnest, something different happened. The rhythm changed. My episodes became very infrequent but also the rhythm changed from the familiar irregular pounding to short episodes of a fast but regular rhythm. Almost as if my heart was trying to repair itself.

I am still not sure what these fast episodes were, whether the a-fib had changed into an atrial flutter or whether it was another form of SVT. Looking back, it was probably the atria remodelling themselves in relation to the positive changes that were taking place in my body. Compared to a-fib they were a walk in the park though, short and sweet!

And then the episodes stopped altogether. The storm was over, and I had weathered it. Even when I came off keto and went back to a normal diet, my heart maintained a normal steady rhythm. A month passed, then six months, then a year, 18 months, 2 years and so on.

Crazy though it seems I even did various "tests" to see if I could send myself into a-fib. I laid off the magnesium for a while, I ate MSG and drank diet soda, drank alcohol, and I even went through a couple of really stressful events and my heart passed with flying colours.

I then pronounced myself cured, not in remission but cured. My doctors had to agree. And life in rhythm is truly liberating. I take no drugs and I have had no surgery. And I'm far from unique.

Over the years I have spent researching a-fib I have come across many, many patients who have rid themselves of this pesky complaint. So don't give up hope if it takes a while to figure out what works for you.

I know how devastating a diagnosis of a-fib can be and I know what it is like to have lived in fear of when the next attack will strike. I consider a-fib to be a wake-up call, a chance to find out what is really going on with your body and put it right. These days I am much more careful about what I eat, ensuring I get good nutrition and the vitamins and minerals my body needs. I watch my weight and drink alcohol in moderation.

I hope you have found my story useful, and that you have taken away something you can use on your own journey. If you have please consider leaving a review for this book so others can find it too.

I wish you good health and happiness.

A-FIB ACTION PLAN

Tackle the big three first. These are the elements which are most effective for reversing a-fib.

1.Lower your blood pressure. Aim for a reading of 120/80 or less, the closer to 100/60 the better.

2. Ensure your blood sugar is under control. Aim for a fasting blood sugar level of less than 100 mg/dL (5.6 mmol/L).

3. Lose weight if you are overweight. A loss of just 10% of your body weight if obese gives you a 50% chance that your a-fib will go away altogether.

4. Get a sleep study if you think you might have sleep apnea.

5. Check for vitamin and mineral deficiencies particularly potassium and magnesium. Consider magnesium supplementation.

6. Overhaul your diet. Avoid sugar, empty calories and processed food as much as possible. Keep a food diary and check for food intolerances.

7. If you are having gastro issues, think about getting checked for h-pylori.

8. Practice good oral hygiene. Get cavities filled and get any gum disease treated.

9. Get your thyroid checked. Thyroid problems are a notorious cause of a-fib

10. Try to avoid stress as much as possible. Learn to actively relax!

Lastly consider getting your c-reactive proteins checked so you can see how you are doing.

Made in United States
North Haven, CT
14 November 2023

44020912R00039